Table of Contents

INTRODUCTION

Maybe someone you know is struggling with borderline personality disorder. The hallmark trait of borderline personality disorder is having a hard time regulating emotions — which can lead to intense mood swings, impulsivity and a number of behavioral problems. Borderline personality disorder (BPD) is one of the most common mental disorders that adults experience. According to the National Alliance on Mental Health, "It's estimated that 1.6 percent of the adult U.S. population has BPD, but that number may be as high as 5.9 percent. Nearly 75 percent of people diagnosed with BPD are women."

How serious is borderline personality disorder? It's very different than someone experiencing some ups and downs in their moods, which is common and can even be considered normal. Borderline personality disorder can be very serious at times, even leading to depression and suicidal thoughts or behaviors, especially in adolescents. People with BPD are also more likely to harm themselves via substance abuse, acts like cutting, and potentially life-threatening eating disorders like anorexia nervosa or bulimia nervosa. In psychiatric settings, as many as 15 percent to 20 percent of all patients are believed to have BPD.

First-line treatment for borderline personality disorder involves therapy, support from family and friends, and, sometimes, medication. There are also many natural ways to help manage BPD symptoms, which include: eating a healthy diet, exercise, many different stress-releiving activities, and supplements that help reduce deficiencies.

CHAPTER ONE

What Is Borderline Personality Disorder?

The definition of borderline personality disorder is "a mental illness that is marked by an ongoing pattern of varying moods, self-image, and behavior."

Personality traits that are common among people with BPD include: anxiety, insecurity and poor self-image, unhealthy relationships, anger, self-harm, and instability. After an event that is upsetting or "triggering," people with BPD have a difficult time coping and calming down (what some refer to as a "hard time returning to a stable baseline"). Experts consider borderline personality disorder to be a "major public health problem" because it's associated with high levels of mental health service use and serious psychosocial impairment.

What are some signs that someone may be struggling with borderline personality disorder? Borderline personality disorder traits include:

Patterns of emotional ups and downs

Impulsivity and being highly reactive

Relationship/interpersonal difficulties

Identity disturbances, including poor self esteem and poor body image

Disturbed cognition

History of the Term 'Borderline' in Borderline Personality Disorder

The term "borderline" was first introduced in 1938 by American psychoanalyst Adolph Stern. He used it to describe a group of patients that did not improve with therapy and whose symptoms did not fit into either the psychosis or neurosis classifications.

At that time, people with neuroses were believed to be treatable, whereas psychoses were thought to be untreatable.

The term was then used to describe people who seemed to exhibit a type of "borderline schizophrenia."

By the 1970s, a deeper understanding of BPD began to emerge. Psychoanalyst Otto Kernberg used "borderline" to describe a personality organization between psychosis and neurosis.

People with borderline personality organization were described as having primitive psychological defenses, which are defense mechanisms to avoid anxiety and are the first to happen developmentally. Examples include splitting, or assigning "good" or "bad" qualities to everything, as well as projective identification or projection, or assigning your negative qualities onto someone else.

The personality organization was marked by instability and issues with one's sense of identity. Soon, a pattern of symptoms began to emerge to describe those with BPD, including:

Unstable self-image: Identity disturbance; can include changes in what they want to do with their lives and what they are interested in

Rapidly fluctuating mood swings: Can range from anxiety and anger to intense dysphoria

Fear of abandonment: Can cause them to cut off people who they fear will abandon them or attach themselves closely to others; may lead to self-harm or suicidal behaviors

Strong tendency for both self-harm and suicidal thinking: Thoughts or acting on harming oneself; could manifest, fore example, in cutting or self-sabotage,

Borderline Personality Disorder Today

Today far more is known about BPD. It's now recognized as a disorder characterized by intense emotional experiences and instability in relationships with behavior that begins in early adulthood and showing up in multiple contexts—for example, at home and at work. In addition, experts have recognized that there is a strong genetic component to BPD.

BPD in the DSM-5

According to the DSM-5, in order to be diagnosed with BPD, a person must meet certain criteria. These include the following:

A pervasive pattern of instability in interpersonal relationships, self image, and emotions

Frantic efforts to avoid real or imagined abandonment

Impulsivity that is self-damaging

Recurrent suicidal behavior or self-harm

Chronic feelings of emptiness

Inappropriate, intense anger

Transient stress related to alterations in reality

Someone with BPD may not experience every symptom. However, according to the DSM-5, a person will exhibit five out of the nine specific criteria listed to receive a diagnosis.

BPD can impact every aspect of your life and leave you feeling out of control. You can experience intense emotions—including depression, anxiety, and anger—that can be difficult to manage. You may question who you are and doubt your self-worth. It might be hard to keep a job or be in a stable relationship.

Living with BPD can be really difficult and feel isolating. However, there is treatment available to help manage these symptoms.

The Ongoing Debate

The term "borderline" has been debated through the years. Many experts have called for BPD to be renamed because they believe the term "borderline" is outdated and potentially stigmatizing. Some believe that BPD should not be classified as a personality disorder, but rather as a mood disorder or an identity disorder.

A 2007 survey also revealed that out of 96 personality disorder experts who completed the survey, only 31.3% wanted to keep the name "borderline personality disorder" in the DSM-5.

Suggestions for the new name have included:

Emotional Intensity Disorder19

Emotional Dysregulation Disorder

Dyslymbia

Signs and Symptoms

The Diagnostic and Statistical Manual, (5th Edition), aka the "DSM-5" that is used by psychologists/psychiatrists, includes a certain criteria/framework that is used to diagnose borderline personality disorder. Diagnosis is based on specific personality traits, signs and symptoms. The DSM-5 states that "The essential features of a personality disorder are impairments in personality (self and interpersonal) functioning and the presence of pathological personality traits."

In the past (as of the year 2000) there were nine symptoms that were used to officially diagnose BPD. To make a diagnosis, someone's symptoms had to include at least five of the following nine symptoms:

1. Making effort to avoid real or imagined abandonment by friends and family.

2. Unstable personal relationships. It's typical for relationship status to fluctuate between feelings of love and hate.

3. Distorted and unstable self-image. Poor self-esteem affects moods, values, opinions, goals and relationships.

4. Impulsive behaviors. These can include excessive spending, unsafe sex, substance abuse or reckless driving.

5. Self-harming behavior, such as cutting or suicidal threats and attempts.

6. Periods of intense depressed mood, irritability or anxiety. These can last between a few hours to a few days.

7. Chronic feelings of boredom or emptiness.

8. Inappropriate, intense or uncontrollable anger. After an angry episode it's common for shame and guilt to be felt.

9. Cognitive disturbances. This can include dissociative feelings, or disconnecting from your thoughts or sense of

identity. Sometimes stress-related paranoid thoughts/psychotic episodes can also occur.

The official borderline personality disorder criteria has changed a bit since 2013. The criteria for BPD now includes:

Significant impairments in personality functioning:
Self identity impairment — Poorly developed, or unstable self-image, often associated with excessive self-criticism, chronic feelings of emptiness, and dissociative states under stress)

Lack of self-direction — Instability in goals, aspirations, values or career plans.

Impairment in interpersonal functioning — having reduced ability to recognize the feelings and needs of others associated with interpersonal hypersensitivity (i.e., prone to feel slighted or insulted).

Problems with intimacy — Intense, unstable, and conflicted close relationships, marked by mistrust, neediness and anxious preoccupation.

Pathological personality traits in the following domains:
Emotional Instability — Unstable emotional experiences and frequent mood changes. Emotions that are easily aroused, intense, and/or out of proportion to events and circumstances.

Anxiousness — Intense feelings of nervousness, tension or panic, often in reaction to interpersonal stresses. Feeling fearful, apprehensive or threatened by uncertainty or losing control.

Separation insecurity — Fears of rejection, excessive dependency and complete loss of autonomy.

Depressivity — Frequent feelings of being down, miserable, hopeless, difficulty recovering from such moods, pessimism about the future, potential suicidal thoughts.

Impulsivity — Acting on the spur of the moment responses.

Risk-taking — Engagement in dangerous, risky and potentially self-damaging activities.

Antagonism and hostility — persistent or frequent angry feelings, even in response to minor insults.

Some experts split patients with borderline personality disorder into four subtypes. Here is a description of the different subtypes of borderline personality disorder:

Discouraged Borderline — Codependent, clingy, go along with the crowd, and really fear being alone or rejected.

Impulsive Borderline — Tend to be highly flirtatious, superficial and energetic. Seeks out attention and always look for the next "thrill."

Petulant Borderline — Unpredictable, irritable, impatient, stubborn, pessimistic and resentful.

Self-Destructive Borderline — Carry a sense of bitterness and engage in self-destructive behaviors.

Causes and Risk Factors

What are the main causes of borderline personality disorder? Like other mental illnesses, BPD is believed to be caused by a combination of genetic, lifestyle and environmental factors — rather than one single cause.

Women are much more likely to be diagnosed with BPD than men. However, some experts believe that just as many men as women are actually affected by BPD, but men may be more likely to be misdiagnosed with post traumatic stress disorder (PTSD) or depression.

Experts believe that factors that contribute to borderline personality disorder can include:

Inheritance, family history and genetics — Research suggests that BPD has strong hereditary links and is about five times more common among people who have a first-degree relative with the disorder. Studies show that there's an estimated heritability of approximately 40 percent among people with BPD.

Early traumatic life events — Examples of trauma that contribute to mental illnesses include physical or sexual abuse during childhood, neglect, death in the family, and separation from parents.

Impairments in brain function — Studies have found evidence of a neurological basis for some BPD symptoms. For example, some investigational studies have found in people with BPD the "emotional regulation system" of the brain doesn't seem to work properly, which affects decision-making, judgment, communication, cooperation and behaviors towards others. There's also evidence of differences in the volume and activity in brain structures related to emotion regulation between people with BPD and those without it.

Is a chemical/neurotransmitter imbalance to blame for BPD? Certain meta-analyses have found that in people with BPD there's "no significant associations found for the serotonin transporter gene, the tryptophan hydroxylase 1 gene, or the serotonin 1B receptor gene."

Can you develop borderline personality disorder at any age? Yes, although BPD is usually diagnosed in young adulthood, such as in someone's teens, 20s or 30s. In most cases, symptoms begin by early adulthood and then remain present in a variety of contexts/situations.

If you have BPD, you're more likely to struggle with other behavioral/mental problems too. This can make BPD difficult to treat, since it can lead to life feeling like it's spiraling out of control. People affected by borderline personality disorder commonly experience symptoms associated with mental health problems including:

Depression

Bipolar disorder (manic depression)

Higher rate of self-harm and suicidal behavior

Anxiety disorders

Substance use disorders

Eating disorders

Things People With BPD Say

Symptoms of BPD are a result of efforts to cope with the constant emotional pain many people with BPD live with.

People with BPD may relate to thoughts such as:

"I have trouble controlling my anger."

"I have trouble maintaining healthy relationships."

"I try anything I can to avoid being abandoned."

"I often feel empty inside."

"I have a hard time knowing who I really am."

"I feel anxious and irritable."

"I engage in risky behaviors that could be harmful to me."

"I think about ending my life."

"I harm myself."

Common Stigmas

People who have mental illnesses often face stigmas, such as beliefs that people with mental illnesses are:

Unpredictable

Dangerous

Ethically flawed

Inferior

Not capable of caring for themselves or others

Unable to integrate into society

BPD is one of the most misunderstood, misdiagnosed, and stigmatized mental health conditions. People with BPD face stigmas such as beliefs that they are:

Dangerous to themselves and others

Manipulative

Attention-seeking

Difficult to work with

Resistant to treatment

These stigmas are not just hurtful, they are harmful to people with BPD, especially when they occur within the healthcare system.

People with BPD experience structural stigma and stigma from individual healthcare providers. One study found that over 80% of mental health staff members viewed people with BPD as more difficult to treat than people with other illnesses.

These misleading and harmful beliefs affect the quality of care people with BPD receive and can lead to:

Poor therapeutic conditions

Premature termination of treatment

Rationalization of treatment failures

Decreased likelihood of forming an effective treatment alliance between caregiver and patient

Emotional and social distancing

Trouble empathizing

Lack of belief in recovery

Negative or inaccurate perceptions of people with BPD

Worsening of the fear of abandonment for the person with BPD

Ways to counter stigma within society and medical/mental health environments include:

Increasing contact between those who have a mental health diagnosis and those who do not

Providing education about mental illness and how to recognize stigma

Discussing experiences living with a mental illness and the stigmas they face

Changing the language associated with BPD

Providing psychoeducation and training to healthcare providers, mental health professionals, and the families of people with BPD

BPD and Other Mental Health Conditions

People with BPD commonly have co-existing mental health disorders, which can mimic or hide the symptoms of BPD and make it difficult to make a diagnosis. These include:

Bipolar disorder

Depression

Eating disorders

Post-traumatic stress disorder (PTSD)

Gambling addiction

Social phobia

Substance use disorders

Tips for Living With BPD

BPD affects many areas of a person's life. Despite the difficulties this creates, there are measures that can be taken to make it easier to manage.

At Work

It can be difficult for people with BPD to gain and maintain employment, despite the desire to work.

A 2019 study suggests that further research into how reducing symptoms, addressing stigma, and increasing support for employment could improve success in the workplace for people with BPD.

A job preparedness pilot project involving a program called "The Connections Place" showed great promise. It was aimed at helping people with BPD overcome emotional barriers to employment and preparing them to enter/reenter the workplace.

Relationships

Relationship difficulties are a hallmark of BPD, but that doesn't mean people with BPD can't have fulfilling relationships.

Early diagnosis and treatment of BPD can help improve the person's ability to form stable relationships.

Therapy that includes partners, family members, and loved ones can help improve relationships for people with BPD.

Therapy that helps people with BPD understand the perspectives of others can also be a way to strengthen relationships.

Self-Image

Internalized stigma can cause people with BPD to feel guilt and shame.

Learning to identify thoughts and emotions, use coping strategies, and understand themselves can help a person with BPD develop a stronger sense of self. This fosters a desire and willingness to engage in the recovery process, and can improve treatment outcomes.

Physical Health

Studies have shown that without adequate treatment, people with BPD are:

More likely to have other chronic medical or mental health conditions

Less likely to make healthy lifestyle choices

In addition to receiving quality treatment for BPD, people with BPD can help their physical health by:

Getting enough good quality sleep

Eating nutritious foods and eating at regular meal times

Being physically active

Keeping track of BPD symptom triggers (people, places, situations, etc.)

BPD by Age

BPD presents across the lifespan and may be thought of in stages:

Premorbid stage (starts in childhood)

Subclinical stage (early adolescence)

First full BPD episode (middle or late adolescence)

Remission and relapse (from middle to late adulthood)

Not everyone with BPD follows this pattern; other trajectories are possible.

Adolescence

BPD tends to first manifest in adolescence. A reliable BPD diagnosis can be made in adolescents as young as 11 years old.

According to the Diagnostic and Statistical Manual of Mental Disorders (DSM-5), the American Psychiatric Association's handbook for diagnosing mental health conditions, BPD can be diagnosed in people under the age of 18 if symptoms are:

Pervasive

Persistent

Not limited to particular developmental stage or a different mental disorder

Present for at least one year13

BPD symptoms can be distinguished from typical adolescent development. Some studies have shown that 30% of adults with BPD report having engaged in self-harm before the age of 13, while another 30% say they started this behavior between the ages of 13 and 17.13

For adolescents without mental illness, impulsivity, identity issues, and affective instability typically diminish over the course of adolescence. For adolescents with BPD, these symptoms tend to increase over time.

Prevalence rates of BPD in adolescents vary widely. Regardless, education around BPD should be given to professionals who work with adolescents, such as youth and social workers, and school health staff.

Adolescents identified as having BPD should always be seen by a healthcare provider to explore their potential suicidal risk, as there are high rates of suicide attempts and completion in adolescents with BPD.

Adulthood

Adults with BPD may see a switch from the symptoms of impulsivity and suicidality predominantly seen in adolescence, to symptoms of maladaptive (negative) interpersonal functioning and enduring functional impairments.

Studies show diagnoses of full BPD generally decreases from young to middle adulthood, but relapse after remission is common.

Older Adults

BPD is understudied in people over age 50, limiting the understanding of BPD in late life. Studies suggest a decline in BPD from middle adulthood to advanced age.

Symptom expression can also change over time. Symptoms such as impulsivity, rule breaking, and emotional turmoil may decline, while symptoms such as fear of abandonment, selfishness, and lack of empathy may remain.

The loss of a spouse/partner or a transition to a nursing home/assisted living facility may contribute to a late-onset exacerbation of symptoms of a personality disorder. This may be related to the loss of social supports which had previously helped compensate for symptoms, and/or a renewed fear of abandonment.

While younger people may self-harm in ways such as cutting, an older adult is more likely to self-harm by refusing food, necessary medication, or medical treatment.

More research is necessary to gain accurate information on the prevalence and presentation of BPD in older adults.

Choosing the Right Provider

It's important to choose a care and treatment provider, such as a therapist, that is:

Appropriately trained in evidence-based, specialized BPD treatment

A good fit for the person with BPD, allowing them to feel as comfortable and trusting as possible

The Four Types of Borderline Personality Disorder

Impulsive Borderline Personality Disorder

Impulsive behavior is a primary symptom of BPD. A person with BPD can act in impulsive and often dangerous ways. They may do this without regard for others or possible consequences.

People with this type of BPD may appear:

Charismatic

Energetic

Elusive or detached

Flirtatious

Engaging or motivating

Some example behaviors include:

Bingeing behaviors: Binge eating, overspending

Risky and self-destructive behaviors: Unprotected sex, sex with multiple partners, driving under the influence, drinking alcohol to excess, doing illicit drugs, gambling

Aggressive behaviors: Outbursts, physical fights, breaking things, hitting things, yelling fits

Discouraged Borderline Personality Disorder

This is also known as quiet borderline personality disorder. People with this type are afraid of being abandoned. They may take extreme actions to prevent real or imagined abandonment.

Compared to people with other types of BPD, people with this type may keep their emotions inside. They also tend to blame themselves rather than others.

Discouraged types may:

Be perfectionists

Be very successful

Be high functioning

Feel alienated and detached in groups

Feel like they don't have real or strong bonds with others

Seek approval but also self-isolate

Engage in self-harm or suicidal behavior

Feel lonely and empty a lot of the time

Signs of discouraged BPD include:
Clinginess

Codependency

Neediness

Anger and emotional mood swings if abandonment issues get triggered

Self-Destructive Borderline Personality Disorder
People with this type of BPD struggle with self-hatred and often feel bitter.

Symptoms of self-destructive BPD are similar to those of other conditions. Look out for these additional symptoms:

An increase in energy

A decrease in the desire to sleep

Feelings of euphoria

These may be signs of a manic episode or bipolar disorder rather than self-destructive BPD. Talk to your doctor so you can be sure to get the right treatment.

Example behaviors of people with this type of BPD include:

Substance abuse: This includes recreational drugs and prescription medications.

Risky adrenaline-seeking activities: People with this type of BPD may do these activities without preparing for them first.

Self-harm behaviors: These may include cutting, burning, scratching, or hitting.

Threats of suicide

Don't discount suicide threats from people with BPD. You may need to intervene and help your loved one get emergency care.

Petulant Borderline Personality Disorder

People with this type of BPD may be angry one moment and sad or sulky the next. They may swing unpredictably between one emotion and another. They may also feel unworthy and unloved. This can lead to relationship challenges and an unhealthy desire for control.

People with this type of BPD can be manipulative. They often feel very dissatisfied in their relationships.

Substance abuse and other dangerous behaviors often follow.

The research literature isn't always consistent about BPD subtypes. Some may list different subtypes or more than four.

Example behaviors of people with this type of BPD include:

Irritability and impatience

Stubbornness and defiance

Passive-aggressiveness

Severe mood swings

CHAPTER TWO

Borderline Personality Disorder Test

Borderline personality disorder (BPD) is a condition that affects a person's ability to regulate (control) their emotions. This can lead to relationship problems and impulsivity (acting or reacting without thinking first).

BPD is diagnosed based on the criteria outlined in the Diagnostic and Statistical Manual of Mental Disorders (DSM-5). This is the standard resource used by healthcare providers to diagnose mental health disorders. Five of the nine criteria must be met in order for BPD to be diagnosed by a mental health professional.

Below is a test with nine questions. If you answer "yes" to a few of these questions, speak to a mental health professional.

Only a trained and qualified mental health professional can diagnose borderline personality disorder, but there are certain questions you can ask yourself if you think that you or a loved one may have this condition.

Border Personality Disorder At-Home Test

Answer "yes" or "no" to the following questions.

Do you have persistent fears of being abandoned?

A person with BPD may make frantic efforts to avoid being abandoned, whether this is imagined or real. They may start relationships quickly and also end them quickly so they don't risk being the one left.

Someone with BPD often shows a pattern of intense and unstable relationships. They may alternate between:

Idealizing: Feeling like they are extremely in love with the other person and even worshipping them

Devaluing: Becoming extremely angry at the other person and hating them

A commonly used defense mechanism in people with BPD involves "splitting." This means they see things as either black or white with no in-between. All of this can lead to behaviors such as ambivalence (being unsure if they like the person or not), avoidance, and extreme attachment in romantic relationships.

An unstable self-image or sense of self is common with BPD. This can affect a person's moods and relationships. Identity disturbance in BPD can cause a person to change their beliefs, behaviors, or values at any time.

This unstable self-image can lead to problems understanding who you are in relation to other people. This can lead to boundary issues in relationships.

Impulsivity or the tendency to do things without thinking first can cause reckless behavior. For BPD to be diagnosed, a person should show impulsivity in at least two areas that are seen as self-damaging. Some examples of impulsivity are:

Irresponsible driving

Spending sprees

Unprotected sex

Could It Be Bipolar Disorder?

There can be overlap between the symptoms of bipolar disorder and borderline personality disorder. If you recognize the symptoms described here, speak to a mental health professional to help you tease out a potential diagnosis.

BPD can result in recurrent suicidal behavior, gestures, or threats. It can also result in self-mutilating or non-suicidal self-injury behaviors such as:

Cutting

Biting

Bruising

Burning

Head-banging

When to Seek Emergency Help

If you have suicidal thoughts, call the National Suicide Prevention Lifeline at 1-800-273-8255 to talk to a trained counselor. If you or your loved ones are in immediate danger, call 911 for help.

Are you highly reactive and prone to rapid and intense mood swings?

BPD can lead to periods of intense mood swings and instability in emotions. Moods may change quickly, often, and intensely. This is called affective instability and causes a person to swing back and forth between:

Dysphoria (dissatisfaction and restlessness)

Irritability

Anxiety

Do you have feelings of emptiness that you cannot shake?

BPD can create a chronic feeling of emptiness inside. This is different from a distorted and unstable self-image. It is also separate from feeling hopeless and lonely.

Some describe it as a lack of self-feeling, while others consider it to be the inability to internalize positive thoughts and experiences.

Problems controlling anger and experiencing intense anger can occur in BPD. Anger is often fueled by:

Oversensitivity

Sudden reactivity

Rapid changes in emotion (emotional lability)

Unhealthy rumination

Decoding Violent Behavoir

Although people with BPD are often portrayed as being violent, they tend to direct negative emotions inward. By contrast, an antisocial personality disorder is characterized by the externalization of emotions and a greater tendency toward physical outbursts.

Do you get paranoid or shut down during stress?

Paranoid thinking can occur, especially in stressful situations, and make a person fear others. Severe dissociative symptoms can also happen. Dissociation refers to feeling you are disconnected from your body, thoughts, feelings, and surroundings. It can also lead to a feeling of being emotionally "flat".

What to Do

If you answer "yes" to a few of the above questions, you should consider speaking with a qualified mental health professional, particularly if any of these experiences are causing you a lot of distress or interfering with your quality of life.

Keep in mind that the results of this test do not mean you have BPD. Only a mental health professional can do a full assessment and make an official diagnosis.

There are treatment options for people with BPD that can lessen symptoms and improve your quality of life. In addition, studies show that the overall rate of remission among people treated for BPD can be high, and symptoms can improve with time.

Borderline Personality Disorder Statistics

If you have been recently diagnosed with borderline personality disorder (BPD), you may feel overwhelmed, scared and alone. But BPD is much more common than you probably think.

Learning the facts about the disorder, including prevalence statistics, can help you feel more empowered to seek help through therapy and support groups. Here are some relevant BPD facts and figures.

Prevalence

In the United States, recent research has shown that 1.6% of the population has BPD.1 That number may seem small, but when you consider just how large the United States is, you may realize that 1.6% represents quite a large number of people.

That percentage means that over four million people have BPD in America alone. While BPD is not as well known as other disorders, it is actually more common than illnesses like schizophrenia.

Gender Differences

Women are far more likely to be diagnosed with BPD than men. In fact, about 75% of people diagnosed with BPD are women; that's a ratio of 3 women to 1 man diagnosed with BPD.1 Researchers do not know why there is this gender difference

It may be that women are more prone to BPD, women may be more likely to pursue treatment or that there are gender biases when it comes to diagnosis. For instance, men with symptoms of BPD may be more likely to be misdiagnosed with another condition like post-traumatic stress disorder or major depressive disorder.

Suicidality

Some of the most sobering borderline personality disorder statistics come from the research literature on BPD and suicidality. About 70% of people with BPD will make at least one suicide attempt in their lifetimes.

If you are having suicidal thoughts, contact the National Suicide Prevention Lifeline at 1-800-273-8255 for support and assistance from a trained counselor. If you or a loved one are in immediate danger, call 911.

For more mental health resources, see our National Helpline Database.

In addition, between 8 and 10% of people with BPD will complete suicide; this rate is more than 50 times the rate of suicide in the general population. Why these rates are so high is currently unknown. It may because people with BPD don't know where to turn for treatment or are misdiagnosed and not treated appropriately.

Misdiagnosis

While 1.6% is the recorded percentage of people with BPD, the actual prevalence may be even higher. In a recent study, over 40% of people with BPD had been previously misdiagnosed with other disorders like bipolar disorder or major depressive disorder.

These illnesses are often cited, potentially because they are more well-known and more easily treated with medications than borderline personality disorder. It's also common for those with BPD to have comorbidities or other illnesses along with BPD.

In fact, as many as 20% of people with BPD have also been found to have bipolar disorder, making their diagnosis and treatment more complicated than treating one disease.

Prognosis

While BPD is a serious mental illness, it is by no means a life sentence. Research has shown that the prognosis for BPD is actually not as bad at once thought. Almost half of people who are diagnosed with BPD will not meet the criteria for a diagnosis just two years later. Ten years later,

88% of people who were once diagnosed with BPD no longer meet the criteria for a diagnosis.

What Is the McLean Screening Instrument?

The McLean Screening Instrument for Borderline Personality Disorder (MSI-BPD) is a commonly used 10-item measure to screen for borderline personality disorder (BPD). Mary Zanarini, EdD, and her colleagues at McLean Hospital developed this paper-and-pencil test based on BPD diagnostic criteria listed in the Diagnostic and Statistical Manual of Mental Disorders (DSM).

There's no biologically based test to definitively diagnose borderline personality disorder; however, mental health professionals often use screening instruments such as the MSI-BPD to help identify the likelihood of BPD and the need for further evaluation and treatment.

Scoring the MSI-BPD

Each item in the MSI is rated as a "1" if it is present and a "0" if it is absent, and items are totaled for possible scores from 0 to 10. A score of 7 is generally considered a valid clinical cutoff, meaning that a score of 7 or higher indicates that a person likely meets the criteria for a BPD diagnosis.1 However, some researchers have proposed a lower cutoff.2

The first eight items of the MSI-BPD represent the first eight DSM-IV/5 diagnostic criteria for BPD, while the last two items assess the final DSM-IV/5 criterion (i.e., paranoia/dissociation).

Reliability and Validity

The MSI-BPD has demonstrated valid, reliable psychometric properties. It has adequate internal consistency and test-retest reliability. It has also demonstrated sensitivity and specificity for detecting borderline personality disorder when a score of 7 is used as the cutoff.

Uses for the MSI-BPD

Clinicians use the MSI-BPD to assess a person for BPD, sometimes in conjunction with other screening tools. Research suggests the MSI-BPD is helpful in detecting BPD in the general population, but more studies are needed.

The MSI-BPD test has been shown to be very effective in detecting possible BPD in people who are seeking or have a history of treatment for mental health problems.

Other BPD Screening Tools

The MSI-BPD is only one of several tools that clinicians use to screen for BPD. Others include the following.

Structured Clinical Interview

The Structured Clinical Interview for DSM-5 Personality Disorders (SCID-5-PD) is an official diagnostic interview from the American Psychiatric Association (APA) that clinicians use to assess for personality disorders such as BPD.

It is an update of the Structured Clinical Interview for DSM-IV Axis II Personality Disorders (SCID-II).4 A mental health professional may use this screening tool to help determine a person's diagnosis by asking questions directly related to the criteria for BPD that are listed in the DSM-5.

This screening instrument also has an optional self-reporting questionnaire with questions, but not all clinicians who choose the SCID-5-PD use this.

Personality Diagnostic Questionnaire (PDQ-4)

The Personality Diagnostic Questionnaire, 4th Edition (PDQ-4) screening test consists of 99 true-or-false questions that can help screen for various personality disorders, including BPD.5

Zanarini Rating Scale

The Zanarini Rating Scale for Borderline Personality Disorder (ZAN-BPD), also developed by Dr. Zanarini, is used for patients who have already been diagnosed with BPD to test for changes over time.

Which Tool Is Best?

A 2017 study comparing correlations, sensitivity, and specificity among the MSI-BPD, PDQ-4, and SCID-II in adolescents and young adults showed they were equally effective in predicting a BPD diagnosis. That said, an older study concluded that the PDQ-4 resulted in a high number of false positives and as a result, the researchers did not recommend its use as a screening tool for personality disorders in clinical practice.

Impact of BPD Screening

BPD is challenging to diagnose and treat, in part because it's often misdiagnosed and confused with other mental health conditions such as bipolar disorder. Further complicating the issue is that BPD often exists with comorbidities, including bipolar disorder, and poses a significant risk of suicide,9 which makes accurate screening tools such as the MSI-BPD particularly important.

Once BPD is diagnosed, however, the clinician can develop a treatment plan to address it. This might include such targeted approaches as dialectical behavioral therapy (DBT), which has been shown to be effective for people with BPD.

Potential Pitfalls of the MSI-BPD

It's important to note that the MSI-BPD is not a diagnostic tool; rather, it's a screening tool that helps determine the likelihood that a person has BPD. An actual diagnosis requires structured and semi-structured interviews and therapy, ideally with a clinician who offers a strong background in BPD diagnosis and treatment. As such, the MSI-BPD is just one of several tools used in the diagnostic process and should not be used alone for diagnosis.

Another potential problem is related to the MSI-BPD's ease of use and availability online, which could allow someone to attempt to self-screen without fully understanding its intent or the implications of the result.

The test is best administered by a professional who can interpret the results and then recommend an appropriate course of action.

Lastly, assessments such as the MSI-BPD provide a picture of a person's mental status only at a particular point in time. Astute clinicians also must take into account the person's patterns of behavior over time.

How to Handle Borderline Personality Disorder in Relationships

BPD is one of the 10 personality disorders outlined in the Diagnostic and Statistical Manual of Mental Disorders (DSM-5). A core feature of this disorder is instability in interpersonal relationships. This can lead to significant challenges in the relationship, both for the individual living with this condition and for their partner.

If you or your partner has symptoms of BPD, it's important that you seek professional help in navigating your relationship with each other.

Effects on Relationships

Research suggests that the attachment style of people with BPD can commonly create difficulties in relationships.

Some issues include:

Fear of abandonmet: This can lead to either becoming overly attached in an attempt to prevent their partner from leaving, or they could choose to leave first before their partner has the chance to leave.

Difficulty connecting: Communication and connecting are challenged by the shifting views of their identity and place in the world. This can lead to difficulty connecting with one's partner and may make the relationship chaotic, feeling like a rollercoaster with many highs and lows.

Mood swings: People with BPD experience instability and reactivity in their mood and tend to view things as all good or all bad. Hostile actions, verbal aggression, and physical aggression may be present.

Distrust: People with BPD tend to be distrusting and suspicious of others. This can cause them to question the intentions of their romantic partner and distrust their behaviors.

One study compared the relationships of couples where one partner had BPD with relationships where neither partner had BPD. They found that the partner who had BPD had a more negative perception of the relationship than their partner, demonstrating that BPD symptoms impacted happiness and trust in romantic relationships.

Supporting a Partner With BPD

If you have a partner who is living with BPD, there are many challenges that can occur, but there are ways you can help support your partner who has BPD and take care of yourself.

These include:

Educating yourself: Learn as much as you can about BPD. Understanding the mental health condition can increase compassion and ease some of the difficulty.

Seeking help for yourself: Get help from a trained mental health professional.

Practicing clear communication: BPD can cause people to jump to conclusions and misunderstand others' meanings. Clearly communicating, and expressing fears to each other can help.

Knowing how to spot symptoms: Save important conversations for when the person living with BPD is calm.

Asking your partner how you can help them: Knowing how to support them when they are experiencing symptoms will help.

Build your own self-care routine: It can be stressful supporting someone with a mental health condition, so building your own social support systems and coping techniques is important.

Borderline Personality Disorder in Men

Signs of BPD in Men

There are notable gender differences in BPD with regard to personality traits, comorbidities, and treatment utilization between men and women.4 Men with BPD are more likely to demonstrate an explosive temperament and higher levels of novelty seeking than women who have BPD.

Comorbidities and Complications

Men with BPD are more likely to have substance use disorders while women with this condition are more likely to exhibit eating disorders, mood conditions, anxiety, and posttraumatic stress disorder.

This may explain why women seek treatment more often, contributing to sampling bias in studies, whereas men are more likely to wind up in prison settings and remain underrepresented in mental health settings.

Substance Abuse

Substance abuse disorders are more common in men with BPD, especially alcohol dependency.6 One review found a lifetime diagnosis of substance abuse in BPD at around 75%.7

Self-Harm

It's approximated that between 60 to 85% of people with BDP engage in non-suicidal self-injury (NSSI).

One study looked at 22 self-harm behaviors in men and women with BPD, and found only two self-harm behaviors are found to be more prevalent in men: head-banging and losing a job on purpose.9 The authors concluded that there may be some gender differences with regard to specific self-harm behaviors, but the majority of self-harm behaviors overlap between the sexes.

Know the Signs of Self-Harm

Someone you know may be engaging in self-harm if they have the following:

Scars

Scratches, bruises, burns

Sharp objects around

Wearing long sleeves or pants

Avoiding showing skin

Anti-Social Behaviors

Men with BPD are also more likely than women to have a co-morbid paranoid, passive-aggressive, narcissistic, sadistic, or antisocial personality disorder. This association with antisocial personality disorder contributes to more men landing in the correctional system rather than mental healthcare settings. One review noted that men more often displayed intensive anger, whereas women more frequently showed affective instability.

Conventional Treatment

There is no official borderline personality disorder test that doctors use to make a diagnosis. BPD is diagnosed by mental health professionals after they carry out a clinical interview with a patient, review their symptoms and medical history, discuss family history of mental illnesses, and sometimes interview family or friends to discuss any relationship and behavioral struggles.

Can you cure BPD? Borderline personality disorder is a condition that can definitely be managed, but will usually stick with someone throughout their lifetime. Symptoms will usually improve with treatment, but can get worse again during very stressful times or if treatment is stopped. To be effective, BPD treatment must also address other existing mental health conditions that a patient's facing, such as depression and substance abuse.

Treatment options for borderline personality disorder can include any combination of the following:

Psychotherapy (or talk therapy), especially Dialectical Behavior Therapy (DBT), which was specifically developed for individuals with borderline personality disorder. (9) DBT uses concepts of mindfulness meditation and acceptance to work through destructive reaction patterns. Another type of therapy that is used to manage BPD is Cognitive Behavioral Therapy (CBT). CBT has the goal of identifying and changing core thoughts/beliefs that lead to problematic behaviors and inaccurate perceptions.

Family therapy or group support may be used. For example, group therapy is a common treatment in the case of substance abuse or eating disorders.

In some cases, use of medications. Because studies haven't shown that neurotransmitter imbalance is a core underlying cause of BPD, medications are not typically used as the primary treatment. However, if a patient is struggling with depression, anxiety or psychotic episodes, their doctor might prescribe medications to help treat specific symptoms. This can include antidepressants such as SSRIs, or selective serotonin-reuptake inhibitors. Medications can be useful for temporarily reducing symptoms like mood swings, insomnia and depression, but they are very unlikely to "cure" borderline personality disorder.

If needed, outpatient treatments, hospitalization or emergency care may be used to stabilize a patient who is experiencing severe distress or suicidal thoughts.

Ways to Help Borderline Personality Disorder Treatment

Therapy or Counseling

Therapy, including DBT, CBT or family therapy, is considered "first-line treatment" for people with borderline personality disorder because it can help to manage destructive thought patterns and behaviors. Psychotherapy takes place between a patient and a licensed and trained mental health care professional who can help point out underlying problems and offer solutions. Sometimes family members (spouses, parents or kids) or close friends may also attend therapy sessions for support.

There are many different types of therapy, and it's common for therapists to combine and adapt elements of different approaches. DBT is popular for treating BPD because it's been one of the most studied types of therapy. In certain clinical studies, DBT has been shown to help reduce suicidal behavior and self-injury, inpatient hospitalization, and treatment drop out better than other treatment options. The most effective DBT approaches include about one hour of weekly individual therapy, a two-hour group skills training session, out-of-session communication as needed, and a consultation between the patient's other doctors and their therapist. Studies have also shown shorter workshops and training sessions (about 90 minutes to three hours long) on different therapy approaches to be helpful for patients with BPD.

Some of the goals of therapy for treating BPD include learning how to better:

Realistically think through perceptions about oneself and others. Therapy helps the patient become aware of ways of thinking that may be automatic but inaccurate and harmful. DBT and CBT are useful for questioning thoughts and understanding how they affect emotions and behaviors.

Interact with others in a way that helps maintain healthy relationships.

Develop skills to better understand how to deal with stress.

Effectively express feelings and emotions.

Control intense reactions to stressful situations.

Reduce self-destructive behaviors, especially substance abuse and suicidal thoughts.

Reduce impulsivity and aggression.

Better-recognize warning signs and plan how to prevent an episode using coping strategies.

Manage mood swings, depression, hopelessness, anger and anxiety. Relaxation exercises, guided meditations, mind-body practices and mindfulness techniques may be used to gain control over stress-induced reactions.

Build skills in goal setting, healthy eating, sleep, exercise habits, and general self-harm avoidance.

If family and/or friends attend therapy sessions, this is helpful for offering emotional support and gaining more understanding, patience and encouragement. Improving relationship skills is important for reducing fighting and anxiety over being rejected or neglected, which is a common trait among people with BPD.

Other types of therapies might be most effective if co-morbidities need to be treated, such as PTSD, substance abuse or eating disorders. For example, DBT plus prolonged exposure protocol (DBT-PE) has been shown to help people with PTSD and BPD, while three-month inpatient treatment using DBT has been shown to help those with eating disorders plus BPD. Other types of therapy that are sometimes recommended for borderline personality disorder treatment include Mentalization-Based Treatment (MBT), Transference-Focused

Psychotherapy (TFP) and Schema-Focused Therapy (SFT).

Help Treat Depression

Some of the most common and concerning borderline personality disorder symptoms are those associated with depression, such as hopelessness, isolation and self-harm. If depression is something you deal with, consider if any of these underlying depression causes might apply to you:

Chronic stress from things such as financial or job related problems

Unresolved emotional problems from childhood

Neurotransmitter imbalance

Hormonal imbalances

Unresolved food allergies

Alcoholism or drug use

Nutrition deficiencies

Lack of sunlight

Toxicity from metals or mold

Identifying factors that contribute to your depression can help you or your therapist to come up with an effective treatment plan. Ways that you can help naturally treat depression symptoms include:

Eating an anti-inflammatory diet (more on this below). Avoid processed foods that can contribute to fatigue or mood swings, including foods with added sugar, sweetened drinks and desserts, fried food, processed meats, refined grains and low-quality dairy products.

Getting daily exercise, especially outdoors. Exercise is a natural mood-lifter and also has anti-inflammatory and pain-reducing effects. Try exercises such as walking, cycling or another type you enjoy for 30–90 minutes daily.

Avoiding alcohol, drug use or even too much caffeine.

Treating nutrient deficiencies, such as vitamin D deficiency, magnesium deficiency or low intake of omega-3 fatty acids. I recommend taking a quality multivitamin, vitamin D3, probiotic supplement, and omega-3 fatty acid supplement daily.

Consider taking St. John's Wort, a natural herb that works in a similar way as selective serotonin reuptake inhibitors (SSRIs) for lifting your mood.

Seek support from family, friends and your community. Find a strong group of friends that you can share your struggles with; joint a support group online or in person; or consider joining a spiritual group or community.

Spend more time in nature. Aim to spend at least 10–20 minutes in the sun daily to lift your mood and prevent vitamin D deficiency.

Anxiety can exacerbate borderline personality disorder by leading to social isolation, difficulties completing tasks, poor self image, use of drugs or alcohol, and so on. Try these remedies for anxiety to help you feel calmer and more in control:

Seek out a therapist who specializes in art therapy, music therapy or mindfulness practices.

Try biofeedback therapy, which helps you relax your body in response to stress/anxiety.

Exercise daily.

Avoid stimulants, including alcohol, drugs and even certain medications.

Take adaptogen herbs, which are a class of healing plants that improve your ability to deal with stress, balance hormones such as cortisol, and help with relaxation. Adaptogens that may help treat anxiety and depression include rhodiola, kava root and ashwagandha, which work by increasing the sensitivity of your neurons, including two important neurotransmitters that regulate your moods: serotonin and dopamine.

Use lavender and chamomile essential oils, which are natural remedies for improving calm feelings and relaxation. You can add 5–10 drops to a warm bath, diffuse 5–10 drops in your bedroom at night to promote sleep, or apply 2–3 drops topically to your skin (such as your temples, chest and wrists).

Create a "bed time" routine to help you unwind at night. If you struggle to get good sleep, natural sleep aids that can help include: making your bedroom very dark and slightly cool, reading something calming, journaling, taking a warm shower or bath with Epsom salts, self massage, meditation, prayer, breathing exercises, taking a magnesium supplement, or drinking calming tea.

Keeping a calendar or daily planner to avoid missing meetings or feeling overwhelmed.

Taking breaks throughout the day to rest, nap or meditate.

Take a magnesium supplement and B-vitamin complex. You can also speak with your therapist or doctor about taking GABA or 5-HTP supplements, which are derived from natural amino acids that support mental health. They have natural calming effects but should not be taken with any prescription anti-anxiety or antidepressant medications.

Lifestyle Changes

Get enough sleep and rest (aim for seven to nine hours of sleep per night) to help prevent fatigue and mood swings. It can be helpful to stay consistent with a regular sleep-wake routine so that your circadian rhythm (or "internal clock") gets more normalized. It's also important to eat a nutrient-dense diet that helps fight depression and anxiety. Whole foods that should be part of your diet to prevent and treat mood-related problems include:

Omega-3 foods, which help to reduce inflammation and support brain function. The best omega-3 foods include wild-caught fish like salmon, mackerel, herring and white fish, walnuts, chia seeds, flaxseeds, natto and egg yolks.

Fruits and vegetables, which increase your intake of antioxidants and vital nutrients that support your mood and prevent deficiencies. Some of the best to include in our diet are: leafy greens like kale or spinach, asparagus, avocado, beets, broccoli, carrots, peppers, tomatoes, mushrooms, blueberries, goji berries, blackberries, cranberries and artichokes.

Healthy fats, which provide important vitamins and minerals that boost energy levels and mood. The best options are: avocados, grass-fed butter, coconut oil, extra virgin olive oil and omega-3s like walnuts and flaxseeds. Avoid consuming trans fats (like hydrogenated oils) and processed vegetables oil, which can promote inflammation.

Clean protein sources, which are critical for supporting neurological function and balancing hormones. The best sources of protein include grass-fed beef, lentils, wild fish, organic chicken, black beans, yogurt, free-range eggs, raw cheese and protein powder made from bone broth.

Probiotic foods that support gut health, cognitive function and production of neurotransmitters. Some of the top probiotic foods include kefir, yogurt, kombucha, miso, raw cheese and fermented vegetables. In fact, a great way to consume probiotics is to drink kombucha every day because it also contains enzymes and B vitamins that boost your energy levels and help to detoxify your body.

As you know Borderline Personality Disorder is a mental disorder and food can contribute to the development, prevention, and management of mental health conditions, depression and anxiety are such mental disorders. So we can say that there is a relation between food and mood.

Our brain always take care of your movements, emotions, heartbeat, your sense and thoughts. it works even while you're asleep.

This means your brain requires fuel to work perfectly and it comes from the foods you eat. So now we are aware of that fact that we can Overcome Borderline Personality Disorder with healthy diet.

Your meal affects your brain because what you eat directly affects the structure and function of your brain and, ultimately, it affects Borderline Personality Disorder.

Food contains various nutritious elements, such as- carbs, proteins, fats, minerals-salts, vitamins and water etc.

A healthy diet is the basic foundation for mental development. Therefore it is necessary for every person to follow a balanced diet chart.

Healthy Diet for People with Borderline Personality Disorder

This situation is difficult for both the patient and the close ones. As a form of treatment, patients are primarily taught to handle emotions. Along with this, counseling of close people is also done.

The help of cognitive behavioral therapy is also taken to connect with relationships.

Psychiatrists also ask questions related to the person's chronic diseases, family environment. This treatment takes a little longer. Although medicines are also given in this, counseling is most important.

Some specialists choose a specific type of therapy, which is called DBT or Dialectical Behavior Therapy.

Here Are The List of Foods That You Can Add in Your Diet

Omega 3 Fatty Acid foods

Omega 3 are the building blocks of the brain and also fat for fuel in the brain that reduces inflammation.

A lot of nutrients are needed to get rid of Borderline Personality Disorder and one of them is Omega 3 and Omega 9 Fatty Acid. It cures from heart diseases to depression.

The needs of our body also keep changing to stay healthy and fit with the time. As soon as we turn 30 plus, our body needs some other nutrients like Omega-3 Fatty Acid apart from nutrients like protein, minerals, vitamins, fiber to stay healthy.

Omega-3 contains alpha-linolenic acid (ALA), eicosapentaenoic acid (EPA), and docosahexaenoic acid (DHA)[3]. It keeps heart diseases away. Keeps blood pressure right. It removes depression, tension and keeps your mood right.

Omega-3 is one such fatty acid that is polyunsaturated fats, which can be taken from food items the body cannot make it on its own. Omega-3 fatty acids cannot be manufactured by the body, so we must include them in our diet.

Foods list that Contains Omega 3 Fatty Acids
Fish

you can get plenty of omega-3 fatty acids from fish. If you are vegetarian and cannot consume fish, then you canalso fulfill the deficiency of omega-3 by taking fish oil capsules.

Flaxseeds

Flaxseeds are rich in omega-3 fatty acids. You can eat these seeds by simply roasting them.

Walnuts

These are the plant based Omega-3s that have a positive impact when consumed. Walnuts is best resource for your diet you can easily take it in the form of dry fruits. It is also recommended to have ¼ cup of walnuts per day.

Peanuts

Omega-3 fatty acids are also found in peanuts. It increases good cholesterol in the body and reduces bad cholesterol.

Chia Seeds

Chia seeds are the best food in your meal. It is rich in omega 3 fatty acids, fiber and protein. It can be consumed by mixing it in smoothies, salad and curt.

Pumpkin seeds

Pumpkin seeds are the good source of omega-3 fatty acids. It also contains fiber and antioxidants. They are good for heart health as well as the brain. Lowers cholesterol and prevents clot formation in the body.

Chocolate

Chocolate is very beneficial for our brain, by eating it, we also get self-satisfaction, which has an effect on our whole body. Eating dark chocolate helps in relieving stress.

It Regulates hormones and reduces stress. Serotonin is found in it. Which Is an antidepressant. Due to the presence of serotonin in chocolate, it keeps our mind fresh and does not allow stress to dominate.

Mediterranean Diet Food

Plant based diet is called Mediterranean diet. it emphasize healthy carbs and healthy fats. Olive oil is the best example of good fats (monounsaturated).

It includes all kinds of vegetables, fruits and grains. Nuts and seeds make this diet better. It is better to cook all your meal in olive oil to grab good fats.

Prebiotic, Probiotic and Fermented Foods

These foods help to heal our gut. Eg:- yogurt, sauerkraut, kimchi, kombucha and kefir. Prebiotics also help to promote healthy gut bacteria.

Foods to avoid in you diet

Highly processed foods change our gut microbiota and can exacerbating anxiety. These are refined foods that tend to lose some or most of their nutrients through processing.

They contain ingredients like preservatives, coloring agents, flavorings, additives (added sugar or salt) and also chemical ingredients which can affect our physical and mental health and should really be avoided.

Alcohol

It reduces the release of serotonin. It also triggers and worsen anxiety and interferes with sleep inflammation.

Caffeine

It can cause jittery sleeping and worse neurotransmitter functioning if consumed in excess amounts.

Refined sugar and added sugar

your brain can be damaged if you add Refined sugar and added sugar meals in your diets,

Refined grains

They can affect our blood sugar negatively.

Processed and fast foods

They basically don't contain any nutrients.

Processed meats

These foods are associated with migraines, mood swings and inflammation.

Artificial sweeteners and food additives

These are associated with headaches, mood disorders, dizziness and migraines.

Precautions

If you know someone with borderline personality disorder who is having suicidal thoughts or thinking of harming themselves, reach out for help right away. You or the affected person can call the toll-free National Suicide Prevention Lifeline (NSPL) at 1-800-273-TALK (8255), 24 hours a day, seven days a week for counseling and help for free.

If you yourself are experiencing any of the following symptoms, consider speaking with a therapist who can help guide you toward treatment and recovery:

Overwhelming sadness or helplessness

Insomnia

Difficulty focusing on work or at school

Trouble carrying out everyday activities

Constant worry

Using drugs or drinking to excess

Feeling very overwhelmed during a difficult life transition, such as a divorce or job change

CONCLUSION

It's important to not get too hung up on the term "borderline." The term is old and may be changed in the future. Instead, focus on working with a doctor or therapist in receiving the proper therapy and getting all your questions answered so that you can manage your symptoms.

BPD is often misdiagnosed because symptoms overlap with other conditions, including bipolar disorder, depression, and post-traumatic stress disorder (PTSD). Thus, the word borderline might more adequately describe the fact that it sits on the border of many other conditions, blurring their distinctions.

BPD is a mental health disorder that affects mood, behavior, and self-image. It typically begins in adolescence, followed by a decrease in symptoms after young adulthood, though relapses are common. People with BPD may face difficulties at work and in relationships.

BPD is often stigmatized, frequently in healthcare. Healthcare workers and mental health professionals should receive training to combat this stigma.

BPD is typically treated with psychotherapy, but medication may be prescribed if necessary.

The better you understand borderline personality disorder (BPD), the better equipped you'll be to manage your condition. Asking the right questions during your conversation will help you know what to expect and how to better navigate your condition

Living with BPD can be challenging for both you and those around you. Know that help is available. Therapy can help you be mindful of your triggers, manage your symptoms, and improve your level of functioning. Talk to your healthcare provider or a mental health professional about which treatment options are right for you.